FROM HOOKED TO HEALED

HOW TO DEFEAT THE ADDICTION MONSTER

T.S. DuBois

T.S. DuBois

INTRODUCTION

Addiction is a challenge that many of us have encountered, either directly or indirectly, with someone we love or know. I personally understand what it's like to live with an addiction and the struggle to break free from something that holds you in its grip. I have overcome several addictions in my life and have learned valuable lessons along the way. Now, I feel equipped with the tools necessary to combat almost any addiction, which is why I decided to compile these insights and share my solutions with others.

One of my addictions was smoking, which is often compared to a heroin addiction in terms of how hard it is to quit. When people asked me how I managed to stop, they often expected a straightforward answer, "cold turkey," or perhaps that I simply used a nicotine patch. The truth is, the process is more complicated than that. I relied on a set of different strategies to help me in my battle.

I wrote this book to provide practical solutions that can help you overcome your own habits. Most habits share common underlying elements that continue to affect us. Our bodies have built-in systems that help us survive, one of which involves dopamine, our feel-good hormone. For instance, when we eat something satisfying or sunbathe, our brains receive a dopamine hit, signaling that this is good for survival. In the past, food was scarce and hard to come by, but today we have access to many indulgences that can trigger a dopamine hit.

In our desire for comfort and stimulation, we have overindulged in modern pleasures. This overindulgence has created internal dependencies that change how our nervous systems function. The natural pathways for reward and motivation have been altered by repeated exposure to excess, causing us to become neurologically attached to artificial highs and psychologically dependent on these experiences.

This book offers solutions and tools to address addictions related to sugar, drugs, social media, shopping, and toxic relationships.

A helpful way to determine if you may be struggling with an addiction is to take a break from the behavior for two days to a week. If you find it challenging to stay away, it may be worth exploring those feelings further. Recognizing this early can lead to positive changes in your life!

T.S. DuBois

TABLE OF CONTENTS

INTRODUCTION ii
CHAPTER 1
    What's the Reason 1
CHAPTER 2
    Support Circle 8
CHAPTER 3
    Spirituality 17
CHAPTER 4
    Obsession 22
CHAPTER 5
    Lifestyle Change 26
CHAPTER 6
    Craving Killer 32
CHAPTER 7
    Consistency 37
CONCLUSION 42
    The Victory Is in the Becoming 42
    Ready to take your healing to the next level? 44

CHAPTER 1

What's the Reason

Before you can begin the journey of breaking free from addiction, you must first uncover the reason you want to quit. This reason will serve as your North Star, the guiding principle you can return to whenever cravings strike, when withdrawals feel overwhelming, or when doubt clouds your progress. Without a clear *why*, the road ahead will feel longer, darker, and harder to navigate. However, with a strong reason, even the toughest moments can be endured because you know what you're fighting for.

The Power of Motivation

Addiction thrives in secrecy, denial, and distraction. It convinces you that "one more time" won't hurt, that you'll quit tomorrow, or that it's not as bad as it seems. Motivation breaks through those lies. When you name your reason, you take control of the narrative, and you begin to reclaim your life.

Your reason doesn't have to be dramatically profound, but it does have to be deeply personal. It must connect with your values, your vision for the future, and the people (or passions) you care about most.

Finding Your Reason: The Pros and Cons Method

One effective way to uncover your motivation is by writing down the pros and cons of quitting. Be brutally honest with yourself. Don't write what you think sounds good, write what's genuine.

Ask yourself:

- Am I quitting to protect my health and live a longer, healthier life?
- Do I want to become a better role model for my children, partner, or loved ones?
- Is my addiction costing me money I'd rather use to build my dreams or support my family?
- Have I grown tired of feeling controlled, ashamed, or powerless?

When you see your reasons in black and white, they become more than just thoughts, they become responsibilities.

Turning Pain into Purpose

For me, the defining moment came after my mother's death. Her battle with cancer, caused by smoking, left me with a bitter realization: I did not want to repeat that part of her story. Watching her struggle and knowing that her addiction significantly contributed to her illness was heartbreaking.

That experience became the driving force behind my decision to quit smoking once and for all.

I hope your decision doesn't come from such a tragic place. But the truth is, many people wait until they've "hit rock bottom" before making a change. Rock bottom doesn't always look like losing everything, it can be a silent breaking point, a realization that enough is enough.

But here's what I want you to remember: you don't have to wait for the worst to happen. You can choose your own rock bottom. You can decide today that you've had enough, and that this reason is your turning point.

Your Reason, Your Anchor

When your addiction monster (cravings) comes, and it will, you'll need something stronger than willpower. Willpower can fade; motivation keeps you anchored. When you feel like giving up, return to your North Star. Write it down. Repeat it out loud. Carry it with you in your pocket or keep it on your phone's lock screen. Remind yourself:

- "I am quitting so I can live long enough to see my children grow up."
- "I am quitting so I can stop handing my paycheck over to my addiction."
- "I am quitting because I deserve to be free."

Your reason doesn't just guide you; it becomes your *why not*. Why not light another cigarette? Because you want to breathe freely. Why not buy another cart of things you don't need? Because you're saving for something that truly matters. Why not give in just one more time? Because your future deserves better.

Multiple Benefits of Quitting

Physical Health Benefits

Improved Energy and Stamina: Quitting smoking, drugs, and sugar improves cardiovascular function and lung capacity.

Better Sleep: Addiction disrupts natural sleep cycles, and quitting helps restore deep, restful sleep.

Clearer Skin and Brighter Eyes: Removing toxins helps your skin glow and reduces inflammation.

Reduced Risk of Chronic Illness: Quitting lowers the risk of heart disease, diabetes, cancer, and liver or kidney damage.

Balanced Weight: Avoiding sugar binges and emotional eating reduces unnecessary weight gain.

Mental and Emotional Health

Increased Focus and Memory: Cutting back on screen time and substances clears mental fog.

Less Anxiety and Depression: Many addictions worsen emotional instability and drain your mental energy.

Genuine Confidence: You no longer rely on outside validation, such as likes or toxic relationships, for self-worth.

Emotional Regulation: You gain the strength to sit with discomfort instead of escaping it.

Stronger Identity: Letting go of toxic attachments helps you reconnect with your authentic self.

Financial Freedom

Save Thousands: Cigarettes, fast fashion, junk food, and impulsive online shopping all drain your wallet.

Invest in Your Future: The money you save can go toward meaningful experiences, education, or savings.

Debt Reduction: Reducing retail therapy and social media-fueled impulses helps prevent overspending.

Spiritual and Personal Growth

Reclaim Control: Addiction takes your power; quitting gives it back.

Deeper Relationships: You attract healthier people when you stop tolerating toxicity.

More Free Time: Without hours lost to scrolling or bingeing, you open space for hobbies and passions.

Greater Self-Respect: Choosing long-term health over short-term pleasure builds discipline and integrity.

Improved Intuition: A calmer mind makes it easier to listen to your inner guidance.

Social and Lifestyle Benefits

Be a Role Model: Show your friends, children, or followers that it's possible to overcome challenges.

Authentic Connection: Real conversations replace empty digital distractions.

Fewer Regrets: Avoid the shame, embarrassment, and consequences that often follow impulsive actions.

Freedom from Manipulation: You stop being controlled by corporations, toxic partners, or substances.

Life Feels More Meaningful: You become present, grounded, and intentional.

Reflection Exercise

Grab a journal and answer the following questions:

1. What is the real reason I want to quit my addiction?
2. Who else in my life will benefit when I succeed?
3. What pain am I preventing by making this choice now?
4. If I continue my addiction, what is the worst-case scenario?
5. If I quit, what is the best-case scenario?

FROM HOOKED TO HEALED

Your answers will become the foundation of your journey. They are the reminders you'll return to again and again, your personal North Star.

CHAPTER 2

Support Circle

Once you've made your decision to quit and identified your reasons, the next crucial step is to find your circle of support. Addiction thrives in secrecy and isolation. It whispers lies like "No one cares," "You can't tell anyone," "Or "You have to do this alone." This is the addiction monster's favorite tactic because the more isolated you are, the more power it has over you.

The truth is, you are not alone. There are countless people and resources ready to help if you're willing to reach out. Support doesn't always look the same for everyone. For some, it comes from family members or close friends. For others, it may be found in a coworker, a counselor, or members of a support group like Alcoholics Anonymous (AA), Narcotics Anonymous (NA), or Overeaters Anonymous (OA). In today's digital world, support can also come from online communities and apps where people share their struggles and victories in real time.

Why Support Matters

Your support circle does more than just cheer you on, it serves three important purposes:

1. **Accountability:** When you know someone is watching, you're less likely to slip. Telling people about your plan creates a healthy kind of pressure.
2. **Encouragement:** When cravings hit, a simple word of encouragement from someone who understands can be enough to keep you steady.
3. **Perspective:** Addiction clouds judgment. Support circles remind you why you started and help you see beyond the craving in front of you.

My Story: The Power of Accountability

For years, I told myself, *"I'll quit smoking on Monday."* Each Monday came, and I failed every time. However, when I finally opened up to those around me about my decision to quit, something shifted. The next time I slipped, I heard the words: "I thought you quit?"

That question stung; it was embarrassing. The dread of hearing those words again pushed me to resist my cravings the next time they surfaced. Accountability may not always be comfortable, but it really works.

Additionally, I spoke with my coworkers who smoked and asked them not to invite me to their smoke breaks. Setting this boundary was vital for my journey. While it wasn't easy, it helped me avoid triggers that could have jeopardized my progress.

Prepare Your Circle for the Journey

Here's the truth: quitting an addiction isn't pretty. In the early days, you may feel irritable, restless, or even angry. Your loved ones might not fully understand what you're experiencing, which is why it's beneficial to prepare them in advance.

Let them know the following:

- You're committed to quitting.
- You might behave differently while your body and mind adjust.
- Their patience and encouragement will mean the world to you.

A simple statement such as, *"I'm sorry if I seem short-tempered, but I'm working hard to get healthy,"* can go a long way in maintaining relationships while you heal.

Modern Tools for Support

Not all support has to be in person. Technology offers many valuable resources:

- Quit-smoking apps that track your smoke-free days, money saved, and health milestones.
- Habit trackers that help you visualize your progress.
- Online forums and chat groups where you'll find people who understand your experience because they're fighting the same battle.

Using a quit-smoking app, I found that tracking my progress was highly beneficial. Additionally, chatting with others who were facing the same struggle provided encouragement on days when my willpower was weak. Hearing from someone who was a week ahead of me offered hope and reassurance that I could reach that point as well.

Building Your Circle

Your support system doesn't have to be huge; it just has to be intentional. Here are a few ways to build yours:

- Tell one trusted friend or family member about your plan.
- Find a mentor who has already walked the road of recovery.
- Join a group (AA, NA, therapy groups, or online communities).
- Set boundaries with people who may unintentionally trigger you.
- Use digital tools to supplement your real-world support.

Smoking / Nicotine	Sugar / Food Addiction
• **Nicotine Anonymous (NicA)** – A 12-step fellowship offering peer support, meetings, and	• **Food Addicts in Recovery Anonymous (FA)** – A 12-step program that helps individuals with

resources to help individuals live nicotine-free.

- **Freedom From Smoking®** – A group-based cessation program offered through community settings, hospitals, and workplaces; participants who join are often more likely to stay tobacco-free long-term.
- **Local support programs** – Hospitals, health departments, and community centers commonly offer smoking cessation and recovery programs.

food, sugar, and carb addictions find recovery through peer support and long-term structure.

- **Sugar & Carb Addicts Anonymous (SCAA)** – Supports abstinence from sugar and refined carbs through a 12-step framework without enforcing strict dietary plans.
- **Online support communities** – Private Facebook groups and online forums provide encouragement, accountability, and shared experiences for people struggling with sugar addiction.

Drugs / Substance Use

Social Media / Internet / Tech Addiction

- **Narcotics Anonymous (NA)** – A well-known, peer-led 12-step fellowship offering structured guidance and emotional support for drug addiction recovery.
- **SMART Recovery** – A secular, evidence-based program that uses CBT and motivational interviewing techniques to support recovery from a wide range of addictive behaviors, available both in person and online.
- **Heroin Anonymous (HA)** – A specialized 12-step fellowship for individuals seeking complete abstinence from heroin and other substances.
- **Internet and Technology Addicts Anonymous (ITAA)** – A 12-step fellowship offering daily online and in-person meetings, as well as multilingual resources, for internet and social media addiction.
- **Media Addicts Anonymous (MAA)** – A structured 12-step group providing practical tools such as media breaks and accountability partnerships for overcoming compulsive tech use.

- **Medication-Assisted Recovery** Anonymous (MARA) – A peer support group for individuals in recovery who are using medication-assisted treatment (MAT).
- **Comprehensive directories** – Organizations like SAMHSA provide online tools and helplines to help locate substance use support groups in your area.

Shopping Addiction / Compulsive Buying

- **Shopaholics Anonymous** – A peer support group modeled after AA that helps individuals address and

Toxic Relationships / Abuse

- **National Domestic Violence Hotline and local DV programs** – Provide confidential support, safety planning, and connections to both overcome compulsive shopping behaviors.

- **Debtors Anonymous (DA)** – Designed for individuals struggling with financial addiction and overspending; it is especially helpful for those dealing with shopping-related debt.
- **Addiction recovery support groups** – Many include sessions that focus on behavioral addictions like compulsive shopping within broader recovery frameworks.
- local and virtual support groups for those experiencing abusive or toxic relationships.
- **Support groups for survivors** – For example, *Survivors Rising*, an eight-week virtual group focusing on boundary building and healing from past toxic relationships.

Reflection Exercise

- Write down the names of three people you can lean on during this journey.
- Next to each name, note what role they might play: accountability, encouragement, or perspective.

- If you can't think of three, list at least one person and identify one online community or app to join.

Final Reflection

The addiction monster wants you to feel alone, ashamed, and powerless. But once you let people into your fight, you cut through those lies. You gain strength, encouragement, and a sense of belonging that makes the journey less daunting with an army at your back. Remember, you don't have to do this alone; you were never meant to.

CHAPTER 3

Spirituality

Spirituality can be a powerful ally in the battle against the addiction monster. Regardless of your specific beliefs, cultivating a sense of faith can profoundly shape your approach to recovery. Many inspiring success stories highlight how individuals relied on their faith in God, engaged in prayer, or practiced meditation to find strength and stability during their journeys. You don't have to adhere to any particular belief system; even embracing meditation or connecting with nature, such as walking barefoot on grass or along the beach, can significantly enhance your commitment to transformation. Being fully present and mindful not only builds inner peace but also empowers you to overcome your challenges with resilience.

Addiction often feels like a spiritual crisis as much as a physical or mental one. It disconnects us from our inner selves, our sense of purpose, and the people and values that once grounded us. This is why spirituality; however, you define it, can serve as a powerful anchor in the storm of recovery.

Whether you are battling addiction to substances like drugs or alcohol, or struggling with behavioral patterns such as compulsive shopping, excessive social media use, or toxic relationships, reconnecting with something larger than yourself can awaken the inner strength you need to fight back. Spirituality does not require religious doctrine or dogma; it is deeply personal and can take many forms.

Faith and Belief: Not Just in a Higher Power, But in Yourself

Many people in recovery attribute their journey to their belief in God or a higher power, which becomes a turning point that helps them stay clean, make different choices, or simply endure another day. Faith gives pain a purpose, adds meaning to suffering, and creates light at the end of what often feels like an endless tunnel.

However, even if you are not religious, faith can still play an important role, faith in your potential to heal, in the process of growth, or in the belief that you are more than your worst mistake. Cultivating a spiritual mindset can help you view setbacks as lessons and relapses as redirections rather than defeats.

"Recovery taught me to surrender what I couldn't control, and that surrender made me stronger." – Anonymous.

Mindfulness, Meditation, and the Healing Power of the Present

Spirituality can also appear through stillness and presence. Practices such as meditation, breathwork, journaling, or even walking silently outdoors can create the mental space needed to understand your cravings and triggers. Instead of reacting blindly, you begin to respond with purpose.

Try sitting in silence for five minutes each day. Focus on your breath and allow your thoughts to pass like clouds. This simple practice trains your mind to stay grounded in the present, where addiction holds less power.

Nature as a Spiritual Practice

For some, connecting to nature is the most honest form of spirituality. Walking barefoot on grass, feeling the ocean's rhythm beneath your feet, watching the sunrise, or lying under a starlit sky can remind you that you are part of something greater. Nature does not judge; it simply holds space for you.

This grounding effect can be especially powerful for those struggling with behavioral addictions like social media or toxic relationships. When the digital world becomes overwhelming or seeking validation feels addictive, the natural world can help reset your nervous system and restore your focus.

Rituals and Daily Practices That Build Strength

Spirituality grows through consistency. Whether it involves morning prayer, evening meditation, writing affirmations, or saying "I am worthy of healing" every time you pass a mirror, these rituals become emotional armor against your addiction monster.

Here are a few simple daily practices you can adopt:
- Light a candle and set an intention each morning.
- Create a gratitude list before bed.
- Repeat a personal mantra when temptation arises.
- Join a spiritual or faith-based support group.
- Take mindful walks without your phone.

The Role of Community in Spiritual Growth

Do not underestimate the power of a spiritual community, whether a church, temple, meditation circle, or a group of friends committed to personal growth. These communities offer accountability, hope, and belonging, all of which are essential for long-term recovery.

Even if you're not ready to share your story, simply being in the presence of people who believe in something can help you find your own sense of belief.

Final Reflection

Addiction strips away meaning; spirituality restores it. It reminds you that you are not alone, not broken beyond repair, and not without purpose. You are connected. You are capable. You are more than your addiction.

With a strong spiritual foundation, whether built on prayer, nature, mindfulness, or belief in something greater, you can begin to rebuild your life, one day at a time.

CHAPTER 4

Obsession

You might be thinking, "This can't be right. I don't want another obsession; that's the problem in the first place." And you're not wrong for thinking that way. Addiction, at its core, is a destructive form of obsession, an unhealthy fixation that hijacks your brain, steals your time, and replaces joy with dependency.

But here's the truth: you can't simply erase an obsession; you have to replace it.

Let's take a look at some of the most successful people in the world, such as singer Beyoncé, renowned for her legendary work ethic and artistry, or the late basketball legend Kobe Bryant, who famously coined the term *Mamba Mentality*. These icons weren't just talented; they were obsessed with their growth, craft, and ability to overcome obstacles. Their focus wasn't scattered; it was intentional, productive, and purposeful. And this, right here, is your key.

Obsess with Understanding: Knowledge as Your New "Fix"

If you're going to beat the addiction monster, you must become deeply curious, even obsessed, with how it works, why it works, and what it's doing to you. Instead of running from your addiction, face it head-on like a scientist, strategist, or detective. You don't just fight it blindly; you study it.

When I was personally battling a smoking addiction, I didn't rely solely on willpower or shame to quit. I dove headfirst into research, wanting to know how nicotine affected my brain, hijacked my dopamine system, and how my body responded to withdrawal. The more I learned, the more I saw the addiction monster for what it truly was, and what it does, which is to feed on manipulation, chemical hooks, and emotional triggers.

Knowledge is the opposite of helplessness; it's power. Understanding creates a shift from being the victim of your addiction to becoming an observer, an analyst, and someone in control.

Turn Withdrawal into a Checklist of Victories

Another game-changer? Studying the withdrawal process itself. Instead of viewing the symptoms of quitting as terrifying or unbearable, reframe them as evidence that healing is underway. Use timelines and resources to know exactly what to expect and when. This gives you a sense of direction and purpose, it's like climbing a mountain, where every mile marker matters.

Here's what this might look like for someone quitting smoking:

Day 1: Cravings hit hard, but they typically pass within 3–10 minutes. You've survived your first wave.

Day 2: Nerve endings start to regenerate. Your sense of smell and taste becomes sharper.

Day 3: Lung function begins to improve. Your body is detoxifying and healing itself.

Week 1: Circulation improves, and energy levels start to stabilize.

Suddenly, every symptom becomes a milestone, not a menace. You aren't just enduring, you're winning.

Redirect Obsession: From Self-Destruction to Self-Discovery

What if your addiction is food-related? Shopping? Social media? Porn? Toxic relationships? The principle remains the same, learn everything you can. What happens in your brain when you scroll mindlessly? Why does your nervous system crave chaos over calm? What reward loop is triggered by that purchase, message, or late-night binge?

When you dive deep into understanding your specific pattern of addiction, you:
- Remove the shame
- Replace confusion with clarity

- Reclaim control from compulsion

Become the Expert on You

Eventually, you don't just become an expert on addiction, you become an expert on what's most important: yourself. You'll know:

- Your most vulnerable times of day
- The emotional states that spark your urges
- Your triggers and escape routes
- What helps you stay grounded

And when you know all that, you've turned your obsession from being stuck in a prison into a pathway toward freedom.

CHAPTER 5

Lifestyle Change

Addiction recovery is not just about saying no to the things that harm you; it's about embracing a lifestyle that promotes healing.

When you're deep in addiction, it's challenging to focus on anything beyond the next craving, the next escape, or the next hit of dopamine. However, as you start to learn about your addiction and uncover its complexities, a crucial realization emerges: this is your chance to reinvent yourself and build a new life.

It's important to recognize that addiction does not exist in isolation. It has become intertwined with your routines, relationships, diet, energy levels, sleep habits, and even your sense of identity. This is why proper recovery demands more than simply quitting the habit; it requires creating a new environment in which the old patterns, the Addiction Monster, cannot thrive.

Lifestyle Change Isn't Just a Bonus: It's a Battle Strategy

Many people view addiction recovery as a battle fought solely in the mind. However, it's equally important to recognize that the body plays a crucial role as well. Your diet, exercise, and sleep patterns are all part of your support system. They influence how effectively your brain regulates key neurotransmitters like dopamine and serotonin, as well as cortisol, the stress hormone. When your physical health is in good shape, your mental health tends to improve too.

This is why quitting an unhealthy addiction, whether it involves smoking, sugar, drugs, social media, or shopping, is an ideal opportunity to adopt healthier habits. Not only do these new habits help fill the void left by your addiction, but they also contribute to a stronger, more resilient version of yourself.

Addiction thrives in chaos, while discipline creates stability.

The Role of Food and Movement in Healing

Let's talk about nutrition and exercise, not as punishment or for appearances, but as medicine.

Food Is Not the Enemy: It's the Fuel

You might be surprised to learn that cravings for sugar, fast food, or processed snacks could actually signal a need for nutrients. For instance, what feels like a craving for cookies may be your body's way of asking for magnesium or leafy greens. By providing your body with better nourishment, your brain will be less likely to push you toward unhealthy eating habits.

If you struggle with impulse control, as many people with behavioral or substance addictions do, maintaining stable blood sugar levels can be very beneficial. Eating balanced meals that include fiber, protein, and healthy fats can help reduce emotional eating, mood swings, and cravings for substances.

"Let food be thy medicine and medicine be thy food." – Hippocrates

Exercise: Your Natural Dopamine Dealer

Here's something I learned firsthand: your brain craves dopamine, and it doesn't care where it comes from, whether it's cigarettes, chocolate, shopping, scrolling, or exercise.

When I decided to overcome my addictions to smoking and sugar, I committed to working out five days a week. My focus was on daily cardio and strength training at least three times a week. It wasn't about achieving a specific appearance; it was about taking back control of my day. This routine provided structure, built confidence, and most importantly, became a natural source of the dopamine my body was desperately seeking.

You don't have to become a gym rat to reap the benefits. The best exercise is the one you'll actually do.

Here are some ideas:
- Dancing in your living room
- Walking your dog
- Swimming laps
- Biking around your neighborhood
- Practicing yoga or Pilates
- Following a 10-minute workout on YouTube

Remember, movement builds momentum. Keep your body moving, and your mindset will follow.

The Digital Detox and the Sleep Connection

Now let's address the elephant in the room: technology addiction, whether that's social media, YouTube, dating apps, or video games.

If you find yourself scrolling into the late hours of the night, feeling numb or overstimulated, you're not alone. But the cost is high. Digital addiction robs you of quality sleep, which makes you more emotionally vulnerable the next day, increasing the likelihood of slipping back into other addictive patterns.

A few tips:
- Set a screen curfew: avoid screens for at least one hour before bedtime.
- Opt for audiobooks, physical books, or meditation instead of screen time at night.

- If you must use devices, consider using a blue-light filter.
- Replace bedtime scrolling with a calming evening routine, enjoy warm tea, dim the lights, or do light stretching.

If falling asleep is still a challenge, consider foods that support restful sleep:
- Red grapes (contain melatonin)
- Pumpkin seeds (contain tryptophan and magnesium)
  - Tart cherries
- Blueberries
- Warm almond or oat milk

Working out in the late afternoon or early evening can also help your body wind down more naturally when bedtime comes. Again, this is where lifestyle habits and addiction recovery work hand in hand.

Let Your New Habits Become Your Healthy Obsession

The truth is, addictions don't disappear, they're replaced. So why not replace yours with something that builds you up instead of breaking you down?

Start tracking your wins:
- The first time you reached for water instead of soda
- That 20-minute walk you didn't feel like taking but did anyway

- That moment you felt anxious but chose a workout over a cigarette

Celebrate your progress not just in recovery, but in the creation of a new you. Over time, these habits won't feel like chores; they'll feel like freedom.

Final Reflection:

You're not just quitting something, you're becoming someone.

Recovery is your blank canvas. A healthier, happier, clearer version of you is ready to emerge. All it takes is the courage to make one better choice... then another... and then another.

CHAPTER 6

Craving Killer

If you've made it this far, you already know that one of the hardest parts of recovery is resisting the cravings. They can feel like waves crashing against you, sudden, powerful, and relentless. The truth is, your addiction monster knows you better than anyone else. It understands your patterns, your triggers, and your weakest moments. It knows exactly when to whisper lies like:

- "You can't survive without me."
- "Just once won't hurt."
- "You'll feel better if you give in."

The addiction monster is clever, but it's not your friend. It's self-serving and doesn't care about your future health, relationships, finances, or happiness. It only cares about feeding itself. That's why you need to be better prepared than it is manipulative.

The Trick of the Monster: False Alarm Mode

One of the most convincing lies your addiction tells you is that you'll die or lose your mind if you don't give in. This is obviously not true. While cravings can feel overwhelming, they are temporary, they come, peak, and pass. Think of them as storms: intense, but short-lived.

Science backs this up. Most cravings last between 3 and 15 minutes. That's it. They feel eternal in the moment, but if you ride them out, you'll discover something powerful: you can survive without giving in. And the more times you do this, the weaker the monster becomes.

Why Lifestyle Choices Matter

Cravings are hardest to fight when your body is worn down. If you're hungry, sleep-deprived, stressed, or dehydrated, your defenses are lowered, and the monster's voice grows louder. That's why lifestyle changes, like eating well, getting enough rest, and exercising, aren't just luxuries; they're part of your armor.

Food for thought: every healthy choice you make sharpens your sword and strengthens your shield.

Your Three Weapons: The 3 Ds

To help you battle the addiction monster, here are three simple, reliable strategies you can use anytime, anywhere. Think of them as your **daily allies.**

1. Drink Water

Thirst is often misinterpreted by the body as hunger, restlessness, or even nicotine cravings. Drinking a glass of water can settle that confusion and give you a slight boost in mood.

- Try lemon water, it acts as a mild appetite suppressant and refreshes your system.
- Keep a water bottle nearby as a physical reminder to sip instead of slip.
- Each sip is symbolic; you're literally washing toxins out of your body and choosing life over addiction.

2. Deep Breathing

Addiction thrives on tension and impulsivity, but deep breathing interrupts both.

- Inhale slowly for 4 seconds, hold for 4 seconds, and exhale for 6 to 8 seconds. Repeat this for 2 to 3 minutes.
- If you smoke, try to shift your focus: instead of inhaling smoke, appreciate the clean sensation of air filling your lungs.
- Over time, you'll notice the difference, your lungs, once deprived, will expand, heal, and strengthen.

3. Distraction

Sometimes cravings can feel overpowering, and simply drinking water or focusing on your breathing isn't enough. In those moments, distraction can be your most effective tool.

- Change your environment: move to a different room, step outside, or take a quick walk.
- Keep a "craving emergency kit": a crossword puzzle, a journal, headphones with a motivational playlist, or even a list of chores.
- The goal isn't to escape, it's to ride out the wave of craving until it subsides.

Distraction works because cravings are short-lived. By shifting your focus, you allow time to work in your favor.

Cravings Are Proof of Healing

Instead of seeing cravings as the enemy, try viewing them as signs that your body and brain are rebalancing. Each craving resisted is a victory, a battle won. Over time, those battles become easier. The monster may scream at first, but eventually, its voice grows faint.

Reflection Exercise:

- Identify your top three craving triggers (time of day, emotions, or situations).
- Next to each one, write how you could apply the **3 Ds** in that scenario.
- Example: *Trigger – stress after work → Drink water + go for a 10-minute walk (distraction).*

Final Reflection:

The addiction monster may know your weaknesses, but you now know its tricks. With preparation, awareness, and the 3 Ds, you possess weapons it can't match. Every craving survived is proof of your strength, and every battle won brings you one step closer to victory.

CHAPTER 7

Consistency

Reaching milestones such as one week, one month, or even one year free from your addiction is a significant accomplishment, and you deserve to celebrate your progress. However, it's important to acknowledge a hard truth: addiction never truly disappears, it lies dormant, waiting for a chance to creep back in.

This is why you must always remain vigilant. The moment you let your guard down; the addiction monster seizes its opportunity. It may not roar with the same intensity as in the early days; instead, it shows up as a whisper, sly, quiet, and unassuming:

- "You've been good for so long; one drink won't hurt."
- "You deserve a reward."
- "You've proven you're in control; now you can handle it."

And just like that, what seems like an innocent decision can reopen the floodgates. The monster smirks because it knows the truth: your brain remembers.

The Science of Relapse: Why "Just One" Is Dangerous

Addiction isn't just a bad habit; it's a rewiring of your brain. When you indulge "just once," you don't reset the clock; you reactivate old pathways that have been waiting for a chance to reconnect.

Think of your brain like a field: the more often you walk the same path, the deeper and clearer it becomes. Even after you stop, the path doesn't vanish, it grows over a little, but the outline is still there. Step on it again, and suddenly it's visible as ever.

This is why relapse can feel so quick and overwhelming. One small step can lead to the whole pathway being reopened.

My Story: The Setback That Taught Me

I learned this lesson the hard way. After making it a month without smoking, I convinced myself I had beaten it. At a social event, I thought, "I'll just have one. I deserve it." That one led to another, and before I realized what happened, I was right back where I started.

The regret was heavy, not just because I had to quit all over again, but because I realized how easily the monster could trick me when I got complacent. That setback taught me a powerful lesson: never underestimate the monster.

Strategies for Lifelong Vigilance

You don't have to live in fear, but you do have to live in awareness. Here are some practical ways to stay ahead of the monster, even after long-term success:

1. Celebrate Without the Substance or Behavior

Learn to reward yourself in ways that don't feed your addiction. Take a trip, buy something meaningful, or enjoy a hobby, **just not the thing you're trying to leave behind.**

2. Stay Connected to Your Support Circle

Don't disappear from accountability once you've had success. Checking in occasionally with a friend, mentor, or support group helps you stay grounded.

3. Know Your Triggers

Stress, boredom, loneliness, and celebrations are common relapse triggers. Recognize yours and prepare for them in advance.

4. Keep Your Tools Ready

Whether it's journaling, exercise, breathing techniques, or apps that track your progress, always have **coping strategies close at hand.**

5. Shift Your Identity

Don't just say, "I'm someone who quit smoking." Say, "I'm a non-smoker." Don't just say, "I'm not drinking right now."

Say, "I don't drink." Your language matters, it strengthens your new identity.

Think of Recovery as Maintenance, not a Finish Line

Recovery isn't a race with a finish line; it's more like tending a garden. You've pulled the weeds and planted seeds of health, but if you stop caring for it, weeds will grow back. Staying vigilant doesn't mean being perfect; it means nurturing your progress consistently so it continues to flourish.

Reflection Exercise
1. Write down one time in your past when you thought, "I've got this," and slipped. What led to that decision?
2. Create a short list of "safe rewards" you can give yourself when you hit milestones without risking relapse.
3. Write a declaration of your identity (e.g., *"I am someone who chooses freedom over addiction."*) and post it where you'll see it daily.

Final Reflection:

The addiction monster is patient. It waits for pride, stress, or celebration to crack your defenses. But awareness is your armor. The fact that you're reading this, reflecting and preparing, means you are stronger than the whispers. Stay vigilant, stay humble, and remember: every day of freedom is worth protecting.

CONCLUSION

The Victory Is in the Becoming

By now, you've done something many people never do, you've started the journey of facing your addiction with honesty, courage, and intention. You're ready to study its roots, confront its lies, and gather the tools to fight back. Most importantly, you've chosen to believe that change is possible and that your future is worth fighting for.

Addiction is not just a habit, it's a learned pattern that rewires the mind, isolates the heart, and hijacks our most precious resource: time. But as you've seen throughout these pages, the very same brain that was once enslaved by addiction can be rewired for freedom. Every craving you've resisted, every trigger you've identified, and every small change you've made has already begun to shape a new path, one rooted in healing, not harm.

You now understand that recovery is not a single decision but a series of daily choices:

- To pause instead of reacting.
- To reach out instead of withdrawing.
- To trade the numbing high for lasting peace.
- To say, "I am more than this."

The addiction monster may roar or whisper, but now you know its voice, and, more importantly, you've found your own: stronger, clearer, and wiser.

Your initial quit isn't the end of your journey, it's the beginning of a life designed with purpose.

A life where your energy is used for creation instead of consumption.

Where your obsessions become passions that build you up, not tear you down.

Where your story no longer revolves around what you're quitting, but around who you're becoming.

So, take a moment to honor yourself. You are not broken; you are rebuilding.

"You are not weak; you are awakening."

"You are not addicted; you are healing."

And healing, true, lasting healing, is the most powerful form of freedom there is.

Final Challenge:

Choose one habit to replace, one ritual to strengthen, and one person to encourage.

Let your recovery ripple outward, Because this world doesn't just need people who've quit, it needs people who've transformed and now light the way for others to follow.

Ready to take your healing to the next level?

Don't battle the Addiction Monster alone—download the Crave Crusher app for daily tracking, motivation, and support on the go. Whether you're resisting cravings, building streaks, or need a visual reminder that you're winning the fight, this app is your mobilized weapon in the war for your freedom. Slay the monster, celebrate your victories, and stay accountable—one tap at a time.

www.ingramcontent.com/pod-product-compliance
Lightning Source LLC
Chambersburg PA
CBHW060507080526
44584CB00015B/1591